D1649077

My Keto Journey

How Keto Dieting + Intermittent Fasting + 6 to 8 Hours of Sleep =

Sustainable Weight Loss & No More Symptoms of Type 2 Diabetes,

Spelling the End to Chronic Disease as We Know It

JOEY JONES

Virginia "Jinks" Jones
(June 10, 1952 - June 1, 2019)

I miss you, Mom.

CONTENTS

ACKNOWLEDGMENTS

I'd like to thank my tiny, but oh-so-important, keto community: Denise Brock, Angela Carr, Amanda & Edmund Gallop, and Michael Poulnott.

Also, I'd like to thank those who have helped me greatly in some way: Bobby "Pabob" Kimbrough, Mitch Kimbrough & Karen Padgett, Joanna Kimbrough Ralston, Connie Carr, Angela & James Carr, Amanda & Edmund Gallop, Denise, Stacy & Mack Brock, Penny & Fran Brown, Tauhwana & Rodney Wray, Paige Janes, Brother Jarrell, Brother Morgan, Sister Amy, Sister Sara, Steve Pinson, Faye & L.D. Burt, Tonya & Brett Johnson, the staff at Encompass, Sonny Fyneface, my lovely sister, Gina, and her daughter, my beautiful niece, Nicole.

There are quite a few others I'd like to thank here—friends, Higdon & Jones kin. I want you to know that I appreciate your phone calls and visits both before and after Mom's passing.

INTRODUCTION

Food breaks down into just three macronutrients. These are fat, protein, and carbohydrates.

We have been taught for more years than I've been alive that the right course to take with our eating is to consume 200 to 300 grams of carbohydrates a day. This has proven to be not only wrong, but to be the primary cause for our health downfall as a society. This 300 grams of carbs recommendation, aka the food pyramid, has led us directly to type 2 diabetes, which then leads us to nearly all other chronic disease that afflicts the American body.

DISCLAIMER

Before I go any further, I should probably tell you these things:

- I hold no degrees, but I am serious in my research and my work
- I am not a doctor, and I am certainly not trying to be your doctor
- If your doctor is not a keto-friendly doctor, then you should probably get another doctor

TRUSTED RESOURCES

When I was out there on the Internet trying to find my way, I ran across so much information. I needed someone to guide me and tell me what was most important.

I got off to a most-excellent start. But then I plateaued with my weight loss. And maybe I got bored. I started exploring the fringes without ever fully comprehending what I was doing and how it was being accomplished. And, not only that, I was starting to have really bad side effects.

Did I immediately get my act together?

No. I remained lost in the wilderness for months.

I am here to save you from having to go through the pain that I went through. I am divulging my secret.

These four doctors offer the absolute-best information that is out there:

- Dr. Sarah Hallberg

- Dr. Annette Bosworth

- Dr. Ken Berry

- Dr. Jason Fung

So, if you wish, you can stop reading this book right now and go straight to my chapter called The Source.

MY KETO JOURNEY

Going Into Summer

Second only to myself, Dr. Sarah Hallberg gets the most credit for turning my life around.

I had been watching tons of YouTube videos on health. Every week or two, I just knew that I had found the answer, that I had unlocked the mystery, and that my health was going to improve. I never lost hope and I always had faith.

And I was wrong every time, until…

Until June 1, 2018, when I stumbled across a TEDx Talk on YouTube given by one Dr. Sarah Hallberg of

Indiana.

She was advocating something called NO GPS, so catchy and memorable a-name. No, not Global Positioning System. But, yes, this one: No Grains, No Potatoes, No Sugar.

I lost about 20 pounds that first month. *The game was afoot!*

That Fall

That fall, I fell in with a bad crowd. They were the cool kids: the smokers, the drinkers, the ones that talk a big game. They were way out on a limb of speculation. And they were so exciting that I never thought to care that I didn't understand what I was doing to my body.

But then the side effects hit.

And I began to see these metaphors for what they really were: chiropractors, who could always go back to cracking backs if they ever lost credibility as nutritionists.

So I wised up and turned to MDs (and MDs only) because they have nowhere to go if they lose their credibility. This proved to be my smartest decision.

Don't get me wrong: I still dip my toe in the waters of chiropractor-turned-nutritionist when I want to liven things up. Those guys spew some exciting ideas.

But they likely ain't gonna give you a rock-solid foundation in how to keep the weight off and how to permanently reverse the symptoms of your type 2 diabetes.

I will attempt to be the bridge between you and the knowledge required for you to stave off chronic disease for as long as is humanly possible.

Enter Winter

Late that fall, I was in a world of hurt.

It was getting cold outside, and cool inside. This slight lowering of the room temperature was having a profound effect on my body during sleep.

See, during sleep, your core body temperature drops. And you combine it with the room-temperature drop and this mystery item—this latter was found to be keto flu—and you have a recipe for uncontrollable, extremely-disconcerting recurring episodes of body shivers. That is what my December looked like.

By January, I had learned that as your body gets rid of

excess sugar on keto, it also gets rid of excess water. And with the excess water goes essential minerals—such as: sodium, chloride, magnesium, and potassium—that must be immediately replenished.

The lady who put me back on solid ground, with this knowledge, was Dr. Annette Bosworth.

That January, I read her book *Anyway You Can.*

And, again, my life was changed for the better.

With Dr. Bosworth came a flood of prized information.

The most obvious: keto reduces inflammation, which rids you of your joint pain. And it works far better than any anti-inflammatory drug on the market.[1]

Then there's the story that she shares about the seizure kids of the 1950s, which still features prominently in my mind. Some of these children were wracked by hundreds of seizures a day. They were put on a strict ketogenic diet and their number of seizures plummeted to zero. Say what?! Also, those children were followed closely from cradle to grave, and they are now dying off. And being autopsied. More surprising findings. They didn't develop cancer. They didn't have Alzheimer's. Their brains were pristine.[2] Whoa, dude! These findings should have set off an atomic bomb's worth of interest in the keto diet. But no. Information of this best kind somehow gets suppressed.

With all of my trials and tribulations, and foolishness, you may be wondering why I stuck with trying to figure out keto. Answer: By the end of January, I had lost an astonishing 60 pounds. And in just eight months.

By February, I had exhausted my resources and had to find fresh ones. A funny man, in the form of an MD doctor from Tennessee, presented himself to me on YouTube. Not only was he a natural comedian, his information was the kind that I was after: that which is unassailable. His name is Dr. Ken Berry.

My MDs led me to the final doctor. Doctor who, you ask? Why Dr. Jason Fung, of course! His book *The Diabetes Code* is easily the best one-stop shopping you could ever possibly think of doing with regard to reversing your type 2 diabetes.

A Bittersweet New Beginning

So, as this body and health transformation of mine occurred, my mom's health rapidly declined. She and I had been on a very tough journey together for nearly 23 years.

That journey came to an end on June 1, 2019. Her passing was about as peaceful as I could have hoped for.

I will miss that woman. Even as a shadow of her pre-accident self, she was still a force of nature. And I loved her dearly.

The day before her passing, my 365 days of being on my new diet were up. The final numbers were in. *I had lost a jaw-dropping 91 pounds!*

FAT

Best Fat

This is, without a doubt, olive oil.

Olive oil will allow you to straddle both worlds. The high sugar one. And the low sugar one, the keto world. And it accomplishes this without any negative impact on the body. How does it perfectly straddle both worlds? By being low in saturated fat.

I recommend that you start with around 6 tablespoons of olive oil per day and slowly work your way up to about 10.

The best-fat list:

- olive oil

Good Fats

Only *after* you've conquered your sugar addiction and reduced your inflammation (by significantly lowering your carbohydrate intake) can you start to ingest copious amounts of good fats (those that are high in saturated fat).

At the risk of repeating myself, I'll re-parrot:

If you've gotten the sugar out of your body, then you can safely consume several or more tablespoons per day, collectively, of these fats: butter, coconut oil, avocado oil, ghee (aka browned clarified butter), MCT oil, bacon grease, beef tallow, and—yes, even the wrongly maligned—lard. These fats are so filling that I wouldn't go higher than six tablespoons per day. But let your personal satiety (pronounced: suh-tie-uh-tee; meaning: that sense of fullness) be your guide.

Reiterating: These good fats may negatively impact your body if you have not given up sugar; reason being that you still have tons of inflammation in your body—*and saturated fat is sometimes unable to safely play in that hostile environment.*

And here's a formalized version of the good-fats list:

- avocado oil
- bacon grease
- beef tallow (aka hamburger grease)
- butter
- clarified butter
- coconut oil
- ghee
- lard
- MCT oil

Note: The good fats tend to have around three times as much saturated fat as olive oil.

Second Note: You may be wondering why avocado oil didn't make the list. You may be saying, "It has the same amount of saturated fat as olive oil," and you'd be right. But, rightly or wrongly, I don't believe the avocado industry to be as tightly regulated as that of olive oil.

Worst Fats

Here are many of the bean- and seed-based oils that you need to steer clear of:

- canola oil
- corn oil
- *Country Crock*® (aka soybean oil)
- *Crisco*®

- *I Can't Believe It's Not Butter*® (aka soybean oil)
- margarine
- safflower oil
- soybean oil
- sunflower oil

The omega-6 to omega-3 fatty acids ratio is disproportionately high in these oils, causing a lot of inflammation in the body. Oh yeah, hydrogenation—*it's a bad thing!*

Fat Summary

The last thing we want to do here is get lost in the weeds.

What am I saying?

I'm saying:

- make sure that you consume mostly olive oil (at least six tablespoons per day)
- that once you're off sugar you can safely consume several tablespoons of good fat per day (examples: avocado oil, butter, coconut oil)
- that you should stay away from bean- and seed-based oils (primary example: soybean oil)

PROTEIN

I basically don't care where you get your protein from. It's all kind of the same. That said, I do have my recommendations in the Grocery-Lists section of this book. But I don't really feel strongly about one over another. I believe you should diversify, eat a great variety.

To me, the most important thing about protein is knowing your number. So that's what I'll share.

Calculating Protein

Take your goal weight in pounds. Subtract 20 from it if you're a man. Subtract 10 from it if you're a woman. Divide that number by 2 and this is the maximum amount of protein in grams that you should have in a day. This will prevent you from losing muscle mass.

CARBS

The maximum amount of Total Carbohydrates allowed per day on a strict ketogenic diet is 20 grams.

I find that I can usually stay in ketosis on 20 grams of Net Carbs per day, which are calculated by subtracting Dietary Fiber from Total Carbohydrates.

GROCERY LISTS

On the pages that follow, I have provided you with three grocery lists. Why? So that you can visualize how I prioritize my shopping. You get to better see what items I see as the essentials.

14-Item Grocery List

Get smart and buy these items only when they're on-sale (buy two of them if it's somewhat non-perishable and you can afford it):

1. avocados (Hass variety; fresh; **perishable**; they spoil so easily, I usually don't buy more than two at a time)
2. broccoli florets (fresh; **perishable**; I alternate between broccoli and cauliflower)
3. butter (somewhat non-perishable; I prefer *Kerrygold* pure Irish butter)
4. cabbage (requires refrigeration, but is somewhat non-perishable when compared to other veggies; lasts at least a week)
5. cauliflower (fresh; **perishable**; likely the only white food that is recommended; I alternate between broccoli and cauliflower)

6. cheese (block, sharp cheddar; somewhat non-perishable, when compared to fresh vegetables; the shredded kind has undesirable cellulose fiber [aka wood pulp] or potato starch in it, which keeps it from clumping)

7. eggs (require refrigeration, but are somewhat non-perishable when compared to other sources of protein; lasts at least a week; pastured are preferred, but any-old egg will do)

8. ground beef (75% lean, 25% fat; aka hamburger meat; **perishable**; look for the label "reduced for quick sale" on the package; if sales are rare in your community, chunk a bunch of these in your freezer)

9. olive oil (*Pompeian* "Robust"; non-perishable; $15 per 68 ounces on Amazon, or wait until there is a sale at your local grocery store)

10. pecans (somewhat non-perishable; I've been able to find them for about $0.75 per ounce; along with pork rinds, they make the perfect keto snack)

11. pepper (*Harvest Farms* black peppercorns with grinder; non-perishable)

12. pork rinds (*Hogs Heaven*; BUY ONE, GET ONE FREE!; make sure they are plain, not BBQ; along with pecans, they make the perfect keto snack)

13. salt (*Redmond Real Salt*; $9 per pound on Amazon; pre-ground fine; non-perishable; I use this under my tongue for an appetite suppressant as I'm transitioning from high-carb back to keto; also, after I'm back into deep ketosis, I take a sip of water from a fresh bottle, put a pinch of salt in it, shake it well, and refrigerate)

14. salt (*Selina Naturally* Celtic sea salt with grinder; non-perishable; I don't know of a more delicious-tasting salt to cook with)

30-Item Grocery List

Get smart and buy these items only when they're on-sale (buy two of them if it's somewhat non-perishable and you can afford it):

1. avocado oil (somewhat non-perishable)
2. avocados (Hass variety; fresh; **perishable**; they spoil so easily, I usually don't buy more than two at a time)
3. bacon (unsweetened; *watch out for hidden carbs!*)
4. broccoli florets (fresh; **perishable**; I alternate between broccoli and cauliflower)
5. butter (somewhat non-perishable; I prefer *Kerrygold* pure Irish butter)
6. cabbage (requires refrigeration, but is somewhat non-perishable when compared to other veggies; lasts at least a week)
7. calf liver (*Skylark*; keep frozen until ready to

use; a slice thaws in just 30 minutes)

8. cauliflower (fresh; **perishable**; likely the only white food that is recommended; I alternate between broccoli and cauliflower)

9. cheese (block, sharp cheddar; somewhat non-perishable, when compared to fresh vegetables; the shredded kind has undesirable cellulose fiber [aka wood pulp] or potato starch in it, which keeps it from clumping)

10. chicken

11. *Chomps* jerky sticks (free-range turkey & grass-fed beef; found at *Trader Joe's*)

12. coconut oil packets (*Trader Joe's*)

13. cucumbers (fresh; **perishable**)

14. eggs (require refrigeration, but are somewhat non-perishable when compared to other sources of protein; lasts at least a week; pastured are preferred, but any-old egg will do)

15. ground beef (75% lean, 25% fat; aka hamburger meat; **perishable**; look for the label "reduced for quick sale" on the package; if sales are rare in your community, chunk a bunch of these in your freezer)

16. heavy whipping cream (causes some kind of unwanted reaction in me; can have hidden carbs and protein because they're allowed to round down the number to zero)

17. hot sauce (*Texas Pete*)

18. macadamia nuts (unsalted; *Trader Joe's*; somewhat non-perishable)

19. olive oil (*Pompeian* "Robust"; non-perishable; $15 per 68 ounces on Amazon, or wait until there is a sale at your local grocery store)

20. pecans (somewhat non-perishable; I've been able to find them for about $0.75 per ounce; along with pork rinds, they make the perfect keto snack)

21. pepper (*Harvest Farms* black peppercorns with grinder; non-perishable)

22. pork rinds (*Hogs Heaven*; BUY ONE, GET ONE FREE!; make sure they are plain, not BBQ; along with pecans, they make the perfect keto snack)

23. salt (*Redmond Real Salt*; $9 per pound on Amazon; pre-ground fine; non-perishable; I use this under my tongue for an appetite suppressant as I'm transitioning from high-carb back to keto; also, after I'm back into deep ketosis, I take a sip of water from a fresh bottle, put a pinch of salt in it, shake it well, and refrigerate)

24. salt (*Selina Naturally* Celtic sea salt with grinder; non-perishable; I don't know of a more delicious-tasting salt to cook with)

25. sardines (watch out for hidden carbs)
26. sour cream
27. spinach (fresh; **perishable**)
28. steak (I go for the tough, yet tasty, $3 cuts; keep frozen; thawing usually takes about two hours)
29. tuna (chunk light in water)
30. yellow mustard (*Heinz*)

74-Item Grocery List

Get smart and buy these items only when they're on-sale (buy two of them if it's somewhat non-perishable and you can afford it):

1. almonds
2. artichokes (fresh; **perishable**)
3. asparagus (fresh; **perishable**)
4. avocado oil (somewhat non-perishable)
5. avocados (Hass variety; fresh; **perishable**; they spoil so easily, I usually don't buy more than two at a time)
6. bacon (unsweetened; *watch out for hidden carbs!*)
7. bell pepper (fresh; **perishable**; is a nightshade; remove the skin and seeds, which can irritate the digestive tract)
8. bok choy (fresh; **perishable**)

9. bone broth (*Pacific*; beef, chicken, turkey)
10. Brazil nuts
11. broccoli florets (fresh; **perishable**; I alternate between broccoli and cauliflower)
12. Brussels sprouts (fresh; **perishable**; in a world without grammar Nazis—another line ripped from Dr. Berry—it's brussel sprouts)
13. butter (somewhat non-perishable; I prefer *Kerrygold* pure Irish butter)
14. cabbage (requires refrigeration, but is somewhat non-perishable when compared to other veggies; lasts at least a week)
15. calf liver (*Skylark*; keep frozen until ready to use; a slice thaws in just 30 minutes)
16. cauliflower (fresh; **perishable**; likely the only white food that is recommended; I alternate between broccoli and cauliflower)
17. celery
18. cheese (block, sharp cheddar; somewhat non-perishable, when compared to fresh vegetables; the shredded kind has undesirable cellulose fiber [aka wood pulp] or potato starch in it, which keeps it from clumping)
19. chia seeds (*Spectrum Essentials*; a great source of omega-3 fatty acids; our ratio of omega-6 to omega-3 needs to be about 4:1, but it's more like 20:1)

20. chicken
21. *Chomps* jerky sticks (free-range turkey & grass-fed beef; found at *Trader Joe's*)
22. coconut oil
23. coconut oil packets (*Trader Joe's*)
24. coffee (*Eight O'Clock* Colombian Peaks, whole bean; I know, a bean is a lectin, which can be a digestive-tract irritant—and my body is certainly proof of irritation and inflammation—but I can't quite give it up; also, the acid sure doesn't help my reflux)
25. collard greens (fresh; **perishable**)
26. cucumbers (fresh; **perishable**)
27. dark chocolate (70% or greater cacao)
28. eggs (require refrigeration, but are somewhat non-perishable when compared to other sources of protein; lasts at least a week; pastured are preferred, but any-old egg will do)
29. eggplant (fresh; **perishable**; is a nightshade; remove the skin and seeds, which can irritate the digestive tract)
30. EVOO (extra virgin olive oil; see *olive oil*)
31. ghee (*4th & Heart* brand; somewhat non-perishable)
32. green bell pepper (fresh; **perishable**; is a nightshade; remove the skin and seeds, which can irritate the digestive tract)

33. green olives in oil
34. ground beef (75% lean, 25% fat; aka hamburger meat; **perishable**; look for the label "reduced for quick sale" on the package; if sales are rare in your community, chunk a bunch of these in your freezer)
35. heavy whipping cream (causes some kind of unwanted reaction in me; can have hidden carbs and protein because they're allowed to round down the number to zero)
36. hotdogs (probably wouldn't be a good idea to eat them every day)
37. hot sauce (*Texas Pete*)
38. kale (fresh; **perishable**; make kale chips in the oven; or heat up a few tablespoons of butter in the microwave and blanch it that way)
39. kimchi (spicy fermented cabbage; *expensive!*)
40. lard (*Armour*)
41. lettuce (iceberg) (fresh; **perishable**)
42. lettuce (romaine) (fresh; **perishable**)
43. *Lite Salt* (for the potassium)
44. macadamia nuts (unsalted; *Trader Joe's*; somewhat non-perishable)
45. MCT oil (*Nature's Way* liquid; somewhat non-perishable)
46. MCT oil (*Perfect Keto* powder; somewhat non-perishable)

47. mushrooms (fresh; **perishable**; starchy, but okay)

48. okra (fresh; **perishable**)

49. olive oil (*Pompeian* "Robust"; non-perishable; $15 per 68 ounces on Amazon, or wait until there is a sale at your local grocery store)

50. olives

51. onions (breaks the below-ground rule, but should be okay in small amounts)

52. pecans (somewhat non-perishable; I've been able to find them for about $0.75 per ounce; along with pork rinds, they make the perfect keto snack)

53. pepper (*Harvest Farms* black peppercorns; non-perishable)

54. peppers (fresh; **perishable**; is a nightshade; remove the skin and seeds, which can irritate the digestive tract)

55. pickles (unsweetened)

56. pork chops

57. pork rinds (*Hogs Heaven*; BUY ONE, GET ONE FREE!; make sure they are plain, not BBQ; along with pecans, they make the perfect keto snack)

58. salmon (wild-caught sockeye is all the rave today)

59. salt (*Redmond Real Salt*; $9 per pound on

Amazon; pre-ground fine; non-perishable; I use this under my tongue for an appetite suppressant as I'm transitioning from high-carb back to keto; also, after I'm back into deep ketosis, I take a sip of water from a fresh bottle, put a pinch of salt in it, shake it well, and refrigerate)

60. salt (*Selina Naturally* Celtic sea salt with grinder; non-perishable; I don't know of a more delicious-tasting salt to cook with)

61. sardines (canned; oftentimes the cheapest have added carbs; I just pour out their sauce and add my olive oil)

62. sauerkraut (fermented cabbage; *Libby's* "Crispy")

63. shrimp

64. sour cream

65. spaghetti squash (a little carby, but a decent spaghetti substitute; serve with alfredo sauce)

66. spinach (fresh; **perishable**)

67. steak (I go for the tough, yet tasty, $3 cuts)

68. Swiss chard (fresh; **perishable**)

69. tomatoes (are a nightshade; remove the skin and seeds, which can irritate the digestive tract; a little sweet)

70. tuna (chunk light in water)

71. turnip greens (fresh; **perishable**)

72. walnuts

73. yellow mustard (*Heinz*)

74. zucchini (zoodle it, and it's another good pasta substitute; dress it in olive oil & butter dressing)

[3] [4] [5]

INTERMITTENT FASTING

Put a pinch of *Redmond Real Salt* (or some other high-quality sea salt) into a sixteen-ounce bottle of water. Shake it up and refrigerate it. After a time, this simple elixir may taste delicious to you.

If you're a sun-up to sundown kind of person, don't eat until at least 10am.

If you're a "vampire nerd" like me (a term coined by a loving cousin, to describe the night-owl behavior of me and another geeky cousin), then you're likely going to have to reinvent the wheel or at least flip the script. And I leave that script-flipping up to you. You've been bucking the system your entire life; you can handle it.

So, back to the 10am thing. I recommend that you go without food and just sip your salted water for as long as you feel good. Bodily. Mentally. I say this because the act of digesting food may actually make you feel worse. So we want to put that off. We don't need to start our day with the negative hit of an insulin response.

If you haven't been strictly keto, you likely won't be able to extend your fast very far into the day. Those carbs will come a-calling.

If you are deep in ketosis, you should be able to make it to at least 2pm and possibly even 4pm. I recommend eating just once a day, at around 4pm. But, nearly as good, is: your first meal at 2pm and your second (and last) meal at 6pm. Then you don't have to worry much about acid reflux during bedtime. Also, don't drink a lot of water at bedtime, or you'll be up peeing all night and you'll be encouraging the acid reflux to flow northward into your mouth.

WATER

I encourage you to get the recommended 8 eight-ounce glasses (aka 4 sixteen-ounce bottles) of water per day. And up to even double that if you sweat a lot and/or are physically active. Of course, each of those sixteen-ounce bottles should contain a pinch of *Redmond Real Salt*. (No, at the time of this writing, I have not asked them to pay me to say that, nor have they offered, nor do they know that I exist.) Another little thing worth mentioning before breaking away to something else: I'm well aware that there are no studies that conclusively show that you should have this or that amount of water; so, I say, let your thirst be your guide, unless it has historically proven itself to be unreliable.

SLEEP

Maybe you're different than me. But probably not so much in this regard.

Me and sleep have had a wicked relationship this past year. Mom was in the hospital four times in those final six months. Because I wasn't trusting enough of the hospital staff, I was there every day that she was there. So maybe you can see how I was getting behind on my rest.

I learned that if I went several days with four hours or less of sleep that my immune system would start to wear down. Also, I would find myself more stressed and suddenly unable to lose any weight.

But if I just got that number up to six, it made a massive difference in my brain function, health, stress, weight loss, and general outlook.

And eight hours is my absolute magic number. See, I can't go higher than eight without my lower back complaining vehemently. But I envy those who can.

JUST THREE RECIPES

Batterless Skin-On Fried Chicken Legs

Ingredients:

1. one family-pack of skin-on chicken legs
2. a few heaping tablespoons of *Armour* lard
3. salt (*Selina Naturally* Celtic sea salt)
4. pepper

Instructions:

Fry skin-on chicken legs in lard on medium to medium-high heat (325 degrees) for 20 to 30 minutes with no batter. Salt and pepper them as they cook. If cooking in a frying pan, turn each drumstick every 5 minutes (to cook the other side). Cover with a lid at regular intervals. Use a meat thermometer to make sure that every piece has reached an internal temperature of at least 165 degrees Fahrenheit. This dish is actually good for you. I fried up an entire family pack and ate off of it for days. It was actually better the second day than the first, and it never made me feel bad. *Kudos to chicken legs!*

Rind Pecan Burgers

This is purely my invention. I am not a big recipe person. I am not on Pinterest. I pulled this recipe right out of my ass. Oooh, nasty! Well, that likely killed our appetites—which just extended our fast. *Win!*

Ingredients:

1. one small package of ground beef (75% lean, 25% fat)
2. one avocado
3. several thick slices from a block of sharp cheddar cheese
4. pecan halves
5. sour cream
6. olive oil
7. salt (*Selina Naturally* Celtic sea salt)

8. pepper
9. *Heinz's* yellow mustard
10.   *Texas Pete* hot sauce

Instructions:

Turn up the heat under your frying pan to medium-high. Make a big, thick burger patty out of your ground beef in the frying pan. Salt and pepper the visible side. Wash an avocado. Remove the skin and seed from the avocado, slice it up, and plate it. Add a large dollop of sour cream to the mountain of avocado slices. I turn my burger, and then salt and pepper everything in the frying pan again. I add three tablespoons of olive oil at this late stage, partly to keep things from sticking. And, lastly, I place in the pan: slices of cheese and the pork rinds and the pecans. When done cooking, mound all this stuff up artistically on your plate and top it off with a few squirts of mustard and decorative drops of hot sauce. You want to talk about a mad kind of delicious. *Oh my gosh-darn hot diggity!* This food is of such a high quality that it deserves its own keto restaurant.

Sunny-Side Cabbage

Now that I've talked about dinner, how's about I get it real backwards and talk about breakfast. Except, thanks to fasting, we missed the first one, so this is actually second-breakfast.

Ingredients:

1. two large eggs
2. a fifth of a head of cabbage (chopped)
3. olive oil
4. butter
5. salt (*Selina Naturally* Celtic sea salt)
6. pepper
7. slices of sharp-cheddar block cheese

Instructions:

Wash that frying pan and fire her up on medium heat. Pour in a few tablespoons of olive oil. Add your chopped cabbage. Salt and pepper it. After about five minutes, flip it. Let the other side brown for about four minutes. Turn the heat down to low. Make some room on the low side of the pan for your eggs. Add two tablespoons of butter to this area. Crack open and add the eggs. Salt and pepper them. Top the hot cabbage with slices of cheese. After a couple minutes, bring the hot cabbage and cheese over on top of the eggs to finish cooking them.

THE NO LIST

One of the core ideas of keto is to kick your addiction to sweet-tasting foods. Then there are those sneaky items that don't taste sweet—such as bread and potatoes—that readily turn to sugar in your body. This should explain why a lot these items made the list. Sometimes items are listed twice, or even thrice, so as to deter the more determined among us from finding a loophole and feeling justified in their bad behavior. If you want to become carb-savvy yourself, just start reading the Nutrition Facts and Ingredients list on the side of every food item. And whenever an item goes over 5 grams of net carbs per 100 grams of weight, alarm bells should sound in your brain. By the way, net carbs are calculated by subtracting Dietary Fiber from Total Carbohydrates.

The No List includes—but is not limited to—the following:

1. agave nectar
2. alcohol (is hard for your body to process and hurts your fat-burning ability, so don't make this a habit)
3. apple fritters
4. apple juice
5. apples
6. artificial sweeteners (acesulfame, aspartame, neotame, saccharin, and sucralose)
7. *aus jus* gravy mix
8. bananas (If I can't have my banana, then where am I going to get my potassium? Answer: avocados, cucumbers, Swiss chard, spinach, mushrooms, Brussels sprouts, and broccoli)
9. batter
10. batter-dipped fish (*Captain D's*)
11. battered fried chicken
12. BBQ corn chips
13. BBQ sauce
14. beans (are lectins, which can cause irritation in the digestive tract)
15. beer (is alcohol and gluten: a lose-lose)
16. biscuits
17. black beans (are lectins, which can cause irritation in the digestive tract)

18. blueberries (12 grams of net carbs per 100 grams of weight; the goal is 5 grams to be keto, lest we forget)
19. bread
20. breadsticks
21. breakfast cereals (e.g. *Apple Jacks*®, *Cap'n Crunch*®, *Cheerios*®, *Corn Flakes*®, *Count Chocula*®, *Franken Berry*® *Froot Loops*®, *Frosted Flakes*®, *Golden Crisp*®, *Honey Smacks*®, *Lucky Charms*®, *Rice Krispies*®... and the like)
22. brown rice
23. brown sugar
24. buns
25. *Burger King*® *Whopper*® sandwich (you could always ask for it without the bun)
26. Caesar salad dressing (aka soybean oil)
27. cake
28. candy
29. candy bars (e.g. *Baby Ruth*®, *Twix*®... and the like)
30. canned fruit
31. canola oil
32. cantaloupe (scores 7 grams of net carbs per 100 grams of weight; just 2 grams from tricking us into thinking it's keto-friendly; there's just one problem: sure it's mostly water, but everything else about it points to it being pure

sugar; there's no fat to speak of and very little protein; remember: a healthy diet is high in fat, moderate in protein, and low in carbs)

33. carrots (at 7 grams of net carbs per 100 grams of weight, they're just a couple of grams away from being keto friendly)

34. cashews (are actually a bean, which are lectins, which can cause irritation in the digestive tract)

35. catsup (better known as ketchup)

36. cereal (aka breakfast cereal)

37. chickpeas (see *garbanzo beans*)

38. chocolate bars (non-dark is the kind you want to steer clear of)

39. chocolate chips

40. cocoa (too carby)

41. coffee (*Eight O'Clock* Colombian Peaks, whole bean; I know, a bean is a lectin, which can be a digestive-tract irritant—and my body is certainly proof of irritation and inflammation—but I can't quite give it up; also, the acid sure doesn't help my reflux)

42. coffee creamer (*Coffee-Mate*®; the Devil. Why? Because it contains corn syrup and soybean oil. *And I love it!*)

43. *Coca-Cola*® aka *Coke*®

44. coleslaw (13 grams of net carbs per 100

grams of weight)

45. *Cookie Crisp®*
46. cookies
47. corn
48. corn chips
49. corn oil
50. *Corn Pops®*
51. cornmeal
52. cornstarch (aka corn starch)
53. corn syrup
54. *Country Crock®* (aka soybean oil)
55. creamed corn
56. creamer
57. Creamy Caesar salad dressing (aka soybean oil)
58. *Crisco®*
59. *Dairy Queen® Blizzard®* milkshakes
60. *Dave's Single®*
61. dessert
62. donuts (aka doughnuts)
63. *Doritos®*
64. energy drinks
65. evaporated milk
66. fast food (basically there's something wrong with everything served: batter, bun, potatoes, soybean oil in condiments, toast)
67. flour

68. French fries
69. fried chicken (battered)
70. fruit
71. fruit juices
72. garbanzo beans aka chickpeas (are lectins, which can cause irritation in the digestive tract)
73. *Gatorade*®
74. grains (remove all from your diet)
75. granola bars
76. granulated sugar
77. grapes (16 grams of net carbs per 100 grams of weight; overshoots being keto friendly by 11 grams)
78. gravy
79. green beans (are lectins, which can cause irritation in the digestive tract)
80. grits
81. high fructose corn syrup (aka HFCS)
82. honey (even the kind grown locally; because, at the end of the day, what honey is first is sugar)
83. honey buns
84. *I Can't Believe It's Not Butter*® (aka soybean oil)
85. ice cream (nope: twice as many carbs as fat)
86. ketchup
87. Lay's potato chips

88.　lemons & limes (6 & 8 grams of net carbs, respectively, per 100 grams of weight)

89.　liquor: vodka, gin, whiskey, scotch, tequila, and Mezcal (see: alcohol)

90.　*Little Debbie*® (oatmeal pie, zebra cake… anything with that branding)

91.　low-fat cheese (cheese where the fat hasn't been messed around with is okay)

92.　low-fat milk (everything low-fat or reduced-fat is bad for you)

93.　maltodextrin (a sugar, frequently used as a bulking agent, that causes more of an insulin response than sugar itself)

94.　margarine

95.　mayonnaise (aka soybean oil; sorry *Duke's*)

96.　*McDonald's*® *Big Mac*® sandwich

97.　milk (I love milk, but my body has told me that it's off-limits, and my research says that the beta-casein A1 protein, contained in American milk, can be inflammatory and may even cause type 1 diabetes; also, there's the issue of lactose [milk sugar]; and milk has been used for time immemorial [at least the past 80 years] to encourage growth by putting a ton of weight on an individual [typically a baby or a football player])

98.　milkshake

99. *Miracle Whip* (aka soybean oil)
100. molasses
101. Mongolian beef
102. monk fruit (is my favorite low-carb coffee sweetener and my favorite brand is *In The Raw*, but it has dextrose or maltodextrin—sugar— in it)
103. monosodium glutamate (aka MSG)
104. *Monster* energy drinks
105. *Mountain Dew*
106. non-dairy creamer
107. noodles
108. *Noosa®* yoghurt (aka *Noosa®* yogurt)
109. oatmeal
110. oats (*Quaker®*)
111. orange juice
112. oranges
113. *Oreo®* cookies
114. pasta
115. pastries
116. peaches
117. peanut butter
118. peanut oil
119. peanuts (are actually a bean, which are lectins, which can cause irritation in the digestive tract)
120. peas

121. *Pepsi*®
122. *Perfect Bar*® (one of my favorite things, but one bar would blow my whole keto budget for the entire day)
123. pie
124. pineapple
125. pinto beans (are lectins, which can cause irritation in the digestive tract)
126. pizza
127. popcorn
128. pop tarts
129. porridge
130. potato chips
131. potato starch
132. potatoes (russet; about 17 grams of net carbs per 100 grams of weight, which puts them about 12 grams away from being keto friendly; they are also part of the nightshade family, which means that that good-for-you part, the skin, is a lectin aka a possible digestive-tract irritant)
133. *Powerade*®
134. powdered creamer
135. powdered gravy
136. powdered mixes
137. powdered sugar
138. pumpkin

139. pudding
140. quinoa (pronounced keen-wa)
141. ramen noodles
142. Ranch salad dressing (aka soybean oil)
143. Ranch mix
144. rice
145. rice flour
146. Rockstar energy drinks
147. safflower oil
148. salad dressings (aka soybean oil)
149. sandwich bread
150. sesame chicken
151. smoking (is one of the very few no-carb "foods" that I absolutely do not recommend; see my section on diverticulitis)
152. soda pop
153. sodas (*Coke*®, *Fanta*® *Orange*, *Mountain Dew*®, *Pepsi*®... all of it)
154. soft drinks
155. soybean oil
156. soybeans (are lectins, which can cause irritation in the digestive tract)
157. spaghetti
158. stevia
159. strawberries
160. sweet potatoes (lots of fiber, but too sweet)
161. sweetened tea

162. sweetened-condensed milk
163. sugar
164. sunflower oil
165. tartar sauce
166. Thousand Island salad dressing (aka soybean oil)
167. watermelon (scores 8 grams of net carbs per 100 grams of weight; just 3 grams from tricking us into thinking it's keto-friendly; there's just one problem: sure it's mostly water, but everything else about it points to it being pure sugar; there's no fat to speak of and very little protein; remember: a healthy diet is high in fat, moderate in protein, and low in carbs)
168. *Wendy's® Dave's Single®* sandwich
169. wheat
170. wheat bread
171. wheat flour
172. white bread
173. white flour
174. white rice
175. wine (dry is better for ketosis than a fruity dessert wine, but all alcohol is hard for the body to process)

These are just some of the food items that impact me personally. I'm sure that I've provided more than enough examples to fuel your imagination, with regard to what your "no list" would contain.

And even this partial list wasn't created in a vacuum. I had some help.

[6] [7]

THE SOURCE

Here's where I provide you with external links, ones that go outside of this book, to those most-valuable resources.

Where to begin, and in what order? Well, at the beginning, of course.

Let's start with Dr. Sarah Hallberg's TEDx Talk on YouTube, published on May 4, 2015:

Reversing Type 2 diabetes starts with ignoring the guidelines | Sarah Hallberg | TEDxPurdueU

https://www.youtube.com/watch?v=da1vvigy5tQ.

Then there's…

- Dr. Annette Bosworth's YouTube channel
  https://www.youtube.com/user/annetteboswo
  rthmd
- Dr. Annette Bosworth's *Anyway You Can* as an
  Audible book, beautifully performed by the
  author herself
  http://a.co/iKV1gxa
- Dr. Ken Berry's YouTube channel; please
  support him on Patreon, so that he can have
  more free time to make his awesome videos
  https://www.youtube.com/user/KenDBerry
- Dr. Jason Fung's *The Diabetes Code* as an
  Audible book, beautifully performed by the
  author himself
  http://a.co/gvLoqTF

GETTING INTO THE WEEDS

I saved this bit of messiness for last, for good reason. I did it because I don't want to make this diet a turnoff.

I know keto to be the most scientific of all diets, which is part of why it has appealed to me so much. But I don't want to turn away those who don't get a thrill from science.

So, my wording has been careful up till now. This book has been my attempt at making keto simple and fun.

But, watch out, I'm about to get all sciency and shit.

Here's some jargon miscellany: sugar in the blood is called glucose; stored sugar—in the liver, for instance—is known as glycogen.

Oh, I'm warming to this. *rubs hands together*

Macros

A really important thing to remember when you're doing this diet: you're never intentionally running a calorie deficit. You are eating meals that are extremely filling, preferably just one or two a day, and those should be tightly spaced (about four hours apart). Your macronutrient aim is for the fat number to account for at least 70% of your calories; protein should come in at around 25%, with carbs at a measly 5%.

Calories Versus Grams

Fat measures 9 calories per gram of weight. Protein and carbs are each 4 calories per gram. This can be a bit of a mindf*ck when you're doing your percentages and you accidentally think about the macros in grams instead of calories.

Calorie Deficits

Running an intentional calorie deficit is likely going to bite you in the ass. See, your basal metabolic rate can shift by up to 40%. This means that if the right amount of calories for you is 2,000 and you only consumed 1,200 that day, then you likely not only didn't lose weight but felt energy-less also. This is because your body's metabolism can pendulously swing in both directions. My suggestion is that you eat one huge meal per day. Or, hit your number. If, for your body type, the recommendation is 2,300 calories, then hit 2,300 as best you can.

People likely don't even believe me when I tell them that I lose a pound a day when I'm doing keto absolutely right. But it's true. And it's just as true now as it was in the beginning.

Important caveat to the previous paragraph's statement: although totally true, this statement is, unintentionally, a bit misleading. Recently, I broke my old rate of weight-loss record: I lost an astonishing 11 pounds in just 4 days. Unbelievable, right? But that was regained weight. I had just gone carb nuts. The inflammation and water weight had returned. So, when I lost all that weight, there was only one pound of new weight loss in that. And then immediately following that incredible weight loss, I plateaued for several days, even though I was still doing keto perfectly. So, I need to be very, very honest and clear here. Let's look at the amount of weight that I lose when I'm pretty serious about keto, which was that 365 days where I lost the 91 pounds. That's a bit under 8 pounds of weight loss per month. Nothing superhuman about that. But it is still really awesome. And you can easily make the same thing happen for yourself. Matter of fact, you can easily improve on what I did.

Struggling to Lose Weight

An unfair yet harsh reality: some of you will do everything right and still struggle to lose weight. The likeliest answer to what is going on is what's called "stubborn liver." The way you fix this is with longer fasts. Two 36-hour fasts per week should take care of that excess glycogen store, by depleting it.

Don't Combine High Sugar and High Sodium

Don't combine a high-sugar diet with one that is also high in sodium. They don't mix. Sodium (aka table salt) has been wrongly accused of being the culprit here. But it is sugar that causes the inflammation, which makes it where the kidneys cannot properly handle the salt, leading to edema (ankle swelling) and high blood pressure (hypertension). So, the answer is simple: kick the sugar addiction, and then you can likely go back to a normal amount of sodium.

Sugar Is Synonymous with Inflammation

Imagine this going on in your blood vessels: inflammation and a thick substance trying to pass through. That's a recipe for a heart attack or a stroke. Sugar is synonymous with inflammation in the body. For as long as you have this inflammation, you do not have a safe space set aside for these helpful guys: saturated fat, sodium, and cholesterol.

Insulin And Cortisol

I haven't really mentioned insulin and cortisol in this book. They are likely the biggest players where your hormones are concerned. If either is significantly high, then you won't lose any weight. Cortisol is the stress hormone and is responsible for fat-storing. There are three relatively easy ways to reduce your cortisol level: more sleep, relaxing walks, and meditation. High insulin levels are directly related to the amount of sugary foods you consume. Eat foods that score low on the glycemic index, and your insulin level decreases.

Autophagy

Our understanding of autophagy seems to be in its early stages. But the gist of it is that it's rapid cell renewal through cannibalization. In other words, a damaged cell is parted out and those bits are given over to a nearby cell that can still be salvaged. Autophagy is achieved with long periods of fasting. It seems that to get the barest minimum result requires about 16 hours per day of fasting. Of course, 20 would get you a bit more. If you regularly fast for 23 hours per day, and multiply that by several times a week, you should see some pretty dramatic age-reversal effects, as I have. My skin cancers on my arms have all but gone away. I had a really bad scrape on the calf area of my right leg. I fasted for 36 hours during its healing process, whereby it turned into gray dust within a week. I brushed the dust away, leaving no trace that it had ever been there. And there was none of the usual scarring.

Most Important Minerals

Here is my list of the most important minerals that a body needs: sodium, chloride, magnesium, and potassium. If you're doing keto, you should keep a very close eye on these. Make sure that the foods you are eating are high in magnesium and potassium. You should be able to easily avoid deficiencies if you are consuming plenty of greens, avocados, and nuts. Also, make sure that you're getting plenty of table salt (aka sodium chloride). And I don't recommend Morton, or any of the other bleached, dried salts. I put *Selina Naturally* Celtic sea salt on my food and a pinch of *Redmond Real Salt* in my sixteen-ounce bottles of water. Works beautifully.

Magnesium

I suffered from suicidal depression nearly the entire time that I looked after Mom.

This is a very difficult topic, but I'm just going to jump right in there as best I can.

About every five years, I'd have a nervous breakdown, which was usually accompanied by a heightened sense of my wanting to kill myself. In an attempt to nip this thing in the bud, I got rid of all of my dad's high-caliber guns, the idea being that I'd just maim myself with a low-caliber one and that should be enough to deter me. And I'm not much of a wrist-slitter or pill-taker. Also, that intense moment would last for only about two minutes, and then I'd have it managed.

Well, bizarrely and unexpectedly, I finally solved this problem back in the fall, when I started taking more magnesium. Who'd have thunk it?

So, now, I not only take a time-release magnesium supplement, but I also take a teaspoon of milk of magnesia every time I wake up wanting to kick, instead of pet, my favorite dog. I also take some extra magnesium when I find myself arguing with people for no good reason.

I find that magnesium not only relaxes, but that it also restores my empathy. It goes a long way toward stabilizing my mood. And it definitely keeps me well away from the edge of the cliff.

Almost-a-Footnote: After Mom's death, I was able to figure out "why" I felt suicidal in the first place. It was because I had built for myself an inescapable prison, one that I had designed, brick by brick, from the ground up, all the way to the heavens. I couldn't live *with* looking after Mom all the time—but what I could live with even less was *not* looking after her. I couldn't bear the thought of putting her in a nursing home, where she would likely be dead in three months. When this lady was the slightest bit under the weather, she required constant one-on-one, 24-hour-a-day, 7-days-a-week care. And, by God, she got it. Me and the few others who helped me made damn sure of that.

No Yo-Yo Here

The yo-yo diet effect does not apply to keto. If you are disciplined in your approach, you will reap the rewards of the keto lifestyle. You will lose weight easily. You'll feel so much better once your body is rid of excess sugar. Your body will no longer require expensive pills, powders & potions[8] (to use Dr. Berry's expression)—and magic dust (to use The Mick's expression)—to prop it up. You top off the approach to your keto diet with 6 to 8 hours of sleep every night—*and you're golden.*

Hunger

As you're keto adapting, or after some crazy carb binge, you'll experience some hunger. Thankfully, there is this awesome hack: put a pinch of *Redmond Real Salt* (or some other high-quality sea salt) under your tongue. And there should be no more hunger or belly growling for a few hours. (The pinch of salt in your water should also help with hunger.)

Antinutrients

Antinutrients are a difficult topic. My favorite one to talk about is avidin. It lives in the white of the egg. It cancels the beneficial effect of the yolk, where the vitamin B7 (biotin) lives. If you've lost the hair on your head, as I have, then you'll want to fry your eggs sunnyside up, in order that you might kill the white and the yolk survive. Another way, albeit more wasteful, would be to just throw away all the whites. I'll rapid-fire some more antinutrient discussion here with... Then there is oxalic acid (found in parsley, spinach & tea and prevents the absorption of calcium), phytic acid (found in nuts, seeds & grains and prevents the absorption of calcium, copper, iron, magnesium & zinc), and glucosinolates (found in broccoli, Brussels sprouts, cabbage, mustard greens, radishes & cauliflower and prevents the absorption of iodine, which negatively impacts the thyroid). And then there is this poorly understood phenomenon: calcium eaten with iron causes the iron to be poorly absorbed.

Fructose And Fatty Liver Disease

Fructose does not get anywhere near the coverage it deserves. It is an even bigger menace than glucose and gets no press. It hides from the glycemic index by not causing an immediate insulin response. But three weeks into eating a lot of fructose-rich food stuff, and you've become insulin resistant and are well on your way to developing fatty liver disease. Luckily, you can easily reverse it, just by cutting carbs out of your diet.[9]

Leaky Gut

Leaky gut is something that has been plaguing me for over a decade now. Maybe even pretty much my whole life. How it works: food containing gluten (prime example: bread) and/or lectins (examples: beans, nightshades) repeatedly irritate the villi (aka the sweeping fingers) in the intestine, causing one or—worse—a whole section of them to atrophy or even die off. Wherever these deaths occur, access to the bloodstream is granted to whole-food particles. This is a crisis of the immune system. The police, the white blood cells, are pressed right up against this area, but they are easily overwhelmed. Because this just isn't supposed to happen. A high-speed chase ensues, and the perpetrator, a bit of tomato skin or seed, finds its way to the Dead End sign (aka the capillaries in the fingertips), and explodes in a fiery crash that goes through the wall (of skin) and emerges on the other side as clear juice. Or at least that's what happens to me.

Water "Hearts" Glucose

Allow me to paint a picture of inflammation in the typical American body. You're being a good American and obeying the food-pyramid guidelines, and you're getting your prescribed 300 grams of carbohydrates per day. All of those carbohydrates turn to sugar, which is known as glucose once it hits your bloodstream. As the overabundance of glucose molecules race along, they each attract hundreds of water molecules. That's where your swelling comes from. And that's why when you get rid of the sugar (aka glucose) by going low-carb, the swelling rapidly goes away. There's no longer an overabundance of glucose there to hold the water in place. And that's why you lose 20 pounds of water weight in the first month of your going keto.

Ketone Urine Strips

Ketone urine strips, which cost around $8 to $10 per

quantity of 100 to 150, allow you to know whether or not your body is producing ketones. Using these strips is typically done early on in your keto journey, when you're still feeling things out and are a bit uncertain about what you're going through. If you pee on a strip and wait 40 seconds, and it remains "beige," then you're still consuming too many carbs. If you pee in the range of "pink" to "dark purple," then you're doing good to great, with regard to your ketone production. This does not mean that your body has figured out what to do with the ketones. But it is a promising start.

Animals Are What They Eat

There's this sensible argument that is being made out there, which says that animals are what they eat. If a cow is fed corn, instead of its usual diet of grass, then it basically becomes a food that irritates the guts in a great many of our bodies.

Antibiotics in Animals

And this also makes good sense: when excessive amounts of antibiotics are given to the animals we eat, microdoses of that antibiotic trickle down to us, get into our gut flora, and kill off our good bacteria, in much the same way as do the antibiotics we take to kill off bacterial infections.

MCT oil

MCT oil is not a gimmick. It really works, providing really quick fuel for the keto mind and body. But it is sort of a rich-person thing. MCT stands for medium-chain triglycerides. The prized acids for ketosis are the ones containing 8 and 10 carbons, respectively. Specifically, these are capric and caprylic acids. What makes MCT oil so special is that it has near-instant access to the liver, where it rapidly metabolizes into ketones. This reserved-and-quite-exclusive HOV lane is called the portal vein, and MCTs have the passcode to it. MCT oil can be found in both liquid and powder forms. The powder form seems to be better tolerated by most. When checking the product description, look for c8:c10. Beware of scams that are only selling you coconut oil, as coconut oil is far less expensive and only contains about 15% MCTs.

BHB Salts

BHB (beta-hydroxybutyrate) salts are another of those rich-person things. It works, but it costs $50 for a half-month supply of the salts. What is it? Answer: man-made (aka exogenous) ketones in a can. It took my body a couple of days to figure out what to do with the stuff—*and not just pee money down the drain.* Lots of keto docs are attempting to cash-in on this craze by coming up with their own blends. And it seems that every blend is using the patented *goBHB®* brand as their source for the ketone salts. Mixed with the salts in the can are essential minerals (e.g. calcium, magnesium, sodium) that are there to encourage better absorption in the body. When buying the stuff, you're looking for there to be 12 grams of BHB salts per scoop.

BHB salts have shown some effectiveness in battling the effects of Alzheimer's. The logic, there, being that the brain has lost its ability to use glucose for fuel—*but what's to say that it can't use a whole new fuel?!* That new fuel being ketones. Well, all I have to say to that is this: taking the salts apparently doesn't do any harm, and it's certainly worth a try. Who wouldn't want one more chance to say good-bye to that loved one who no longer remembers them? I would.

I tried the *Ignite Keto* brand, by the way, and it was fine.

Walking to Lose Weight Doesn't Work

Walking to lose weight does not work in most cases. Success has to do with how consistent and vigorous you are with the routine. Most people just aren't going at it hard enough and end up burning fewer than 10% of the calories they consume. For the first six months of my diet, I just so happened to not exercise one bit. I still lost nearly 50 pounds. It was around that time that I had this conscious thought: let's see if I can lose the whole hundred pounds without hitting a lick at exercise. And that's how I lost 91 pounds in exactly one year: by not exercising. I am not advocating that you do not exercise. Brisk walking for 30 minutes is great for cardio and relaxation. So I'm not knocking it. I'm just pointing out that it shouldn't be a part of your weight-loss strategy. The weight loss will be achieved through changes in your diet, and that alone.[10]

Multi-Functional Meter

After about six months of doing keto, you may want to up your game. I did. I felt that I'd kicked type 2 diabetes, but I was still having episodes of brain fog and periods where I wasn't losing weight (aka plateaued). I decided that I wanted to put an end to the guessing and to have a greater understanding of my body. I needed a meter that would check both my blood glucose and my blood ketones, almost simultaneously. I went with Dr. Bosworth's recommendation and have not regretted my choice. The device is put out by *ForaCare*. And, at the time of this writing, it's the multi-functional *Fora 6 Connect*, which costs $110 and comes with 50 of each kind of strip, a lancing device, and 100 lancets.

For the first week, I tested myself every day. After that, I would only test myself when I felt really bad or really good. One day, I felt especially good. I had fasted for far more than the 8-hour minimum. My blood glucose came in at 75, and my blood-ketone number was 3.0. Diabetics might would be a little alarmed by that blood-sugar number, saying that it's "spooky" low. But when you're deep in ketosis, and your blood sugar is rock-solid stable, that "75" is the absolute perfect number. Now, to translate the second number. And, to do this, I will borrow from Dr. Bosworth's book…

Blood Ketones

Understanding what your blood-ketone number means:[11]

- "Nutritional ketosis" begins at 0.5 millimoles per liter (mmol/L) of beta-hydroxybutyrate (BHB)
- "Optimal Zone" is 1.8
- "Fasting Ketosis" is 3.5
- "Starvation Ketosis" is 7.0
- And "Ketoacidosis" is 10

Blood Glucose

Understanding what your fasting blood-glucose number means:

- if, after 8 hours of fasting (aka a good night's sleep), your blood glucose measures under 100 milligrams per deciliter (mg/dL), then you're considered "normal"
- 100 to 124, and you're "prediabetic"
- 125 and higher, and you're "diabetic"

Ketosis Versus Ketoacidosis

People oftentimes confuse keto with ketoacidosis. Keto is short for ketosis (a normal process where your body doesn't have enough carbs for fuel and instead burns fat to make ketones for energy) and not the latter. The latter, ketoacidosis, occurs in those who have type 1 diabetes. They are dehydrated, producing way too many ketones, and are unable to produce enough insulin. They can become violently ill and may even die.

A1C

An A1C (glycated hemoglobin) test reflects your average blood glucose levels over the past three months and is another way of checking for diabetes. Here's how the numbers break down:

- below 5.7%, and you're considered "normal"
- between 5.7% and 6.4%, and you're "prediabetic"
- test twice at 6.5% and higher, and you're "diabetic"

Diverticulitis

Switching gears now to a hot-button topic that is filled with denial (aka Da Nile) and makes dramatists of those who don't even care for theatrics. Yeah, you guessed it. I'm referring to those little pouches that form on your colon (aka large intestine). Seeds, nuts, and popcorn are neither the cause of diverticulosis (the condition) nor diverticulitis (the flare-up). This is a medical lie that has propagated throughout our society, and is even spread by doctors today. A 2008 JAMA study, which involved over 10,000 patients, showed that the actual things that put you at increased risk for diverticulosis and diverticulitis are the following: being overweight, consuming processed meats (the grainless, mushy stuff), and smoking. Sorry smokers. Now, please, go back to eating your seeds and nuts. Maybe ease up on the popcorn though, as it's corn.[12]

Neti Pot

I am a huge proponent of the neti pot. Maybe it's because it's an effective method of treating the after-effects of my acid reflux. Anyway, I have this amazing kit that's put out by *Himalayan Chandra*, which includes an amazingly-designed ceramic neti pot, a 2-oz bottle of *Neti Wash Plus*, and a 10-oz jar of 99.99% USP grade salt, all for less than $25. I've been using this set-up for three years now, with great success. I no longer get nasal/sinus infections. For preventive maintenance, I do the neti-pot thing about two or three times a week.

Please read and follow the instructions that come with your pot. I do the following:

1. Bring a quart of clean water (filtered, spring, or purified) to a boil (takes about 10 minutes)
2. Let stand for 10 minutes, and then (without scalding yourself) pour hot water into and all over your neti pot, which is already clean but has been in storage for more than a minute
3. Let the water in the boiler stand for about 20 more minutes, until it is warm (but not hot) when poured over the tender flesh of the forearm—*it is now ready for use!*
4. Add a level scoop of neti salt from the isotonic

(shallow) side of the special double-sided spoon to the neti pot

5. Add a couple of drops of *Neti Wash Plus* to the neti pot (this step is nice, but not absolutely necessary)

6. Fill the neti pot, full, with water from your boiler

7. Over a sink, with your mouth hanging open and your head tilted to one side, connect the spout of the neti pot to your upper nostril and pour until the pot is empty

8. Repeat Steps 4, 5 & 6 (re-adding salt, drops of neti wash, and water to your pot)

9. Turn on your faucet to where, after you've finished your neti-pot treatment, the water will be very warm; also, turn on the stove-top eye, again, and start bringing the remaining water back to a boil

10. Repeat Step 7 (connecting the neti-pot spout to your other nostril and pouring until empty)

11. Wash your hands with dishwashing detergent

12. Turn off the re-boiled water

13. Use your clean hands, running warm water, and additional dishwashing detergent to thoroughly wash your neti pot, both inside and out

14. Finally, use the freshly re-boiled water, while still hot, to re-sterilize your neti pot

15. Anticlimactically, invert your clean neti pot in the draining board and allow it to air dry

16. *Sike!* You're still going to have to do the drain-your-nose thing over the trashcan: bend at the waist over the biggest trashcan in your house and tilt your head to one side; after a few moments, some salty water and stringy snot should start to flow from your lower nostril; don't be alarmed; allow the nostril to finish draining, and then tilt your head to the opposite side and give the other nostril an opportunity to drain

17. Lastly, before going out in public, wash your face and lightly blow your nose into a tissue

Note: After all that, you may still have some salty water and stringy snot drain down your throat, especially when you lay down. As you might already have suspected, this is perfectly normal.

One of the main things about the neti pot for me is its cleanliness. If you're not a clean freak, you may not want to do this. A few people have reportedly contracted a fatal brain infection from improper neti-pot use, which was caused by a Pac-Man-like amoeba (where your brain is the pellets and your soul… the ghosts). This infection is believed to be a result of using water that had not been properly sterilized or a pot that had not been properly cleaned.

BPA

Bisphenol A, better known as BPA, is a plastic used to line metal cans and has been used to make water bottles and other kitchen items. It has been shown to be able to penetrate cell walls and is believed to be very toxic to humans. Because of BPA water pollution, sea salt mined from ancient seas, which are usually hundreds of miles inland, is preferable to that which is harvested from "living seas," ones that are currently being sailed and otherwise trafficked.

How I Weigh in the Morning

I'm sure this will sound like something unimportant. Or, worse, psycho-mumbo-jumbo. But it's been an effective mind game both times that I've had success losing a lot of weight.

So, here goes the explanation (and take it for what it's worth to you):

When I wake up in the morning, I don't take a sip of water. Instead, I hop out of bed, put on a minimal amount of clothing (just shoes, underwear, and a t-shirt), and then I go relieve myself (urinate and have a big, juicy bowel movement).

Sometimes, I have to walk around a bit before the BM will come. I'm patient. I still don't take a sip from that bottle of water.

The timing of the bowel movements didn't happen by accident. I trained myself to go at this psychologically-important part of the day: knowing that there's the possibility that you're going to offload a lot of weight every morning really gives you something to look forward to on your weight-loss journey.

So, now that we're a pound lighter, it's time to weigh in.

I already know how much my shirt, shoes, and drawers add to me, so I perform the easy mental calculation—*and get my naked weight.* That deduction for clothing amounts to either two or three pounds, depending on the type of shoes I'm wearing (loafers or jogging shoes).

I also have various gear-configuration deductions: blue jeans (add 2 pounds), keys, box-cutter knife, smartphone, wallet, ball cap. *Oh, man! All this stuff could add up to four, five, and—even—six pounds, back when I wore "circus tents" for clothes!*

Oh yeah, I almost forgot, I'm a round-downer (just like your Nutrition Facts folks) when it comes to recording my weight. Don't know exactly why that little detail has proven itself to be so damned important, except—*duh!*—it lifts the spirits a wee bit on those disheartened days.

There Is No "Essential" Carb

There is no such thing as an essential carbohydrate. This is extremely important for you to take to heart—*and believe!* And, whether you believe it or not, it's a fact. It's kind of like gravity that way: you don't just float off into space on that same day you become a flat-earther.

On the other hand, there are essential fats (aka fatty acids) that your body must have. If enough time goes by where you're not getting them, you will get sick and die. There are also essential proteins (aka amino acids), where if you don't get them for a long enough period of time—you guessed it—*you die!*

But there is no essential carbohydrate: no essential starch, no essential sugar.[13]

94

And, with that, I hope that I've won you over to low-carb, which is the foundation of keto. Going low-carb is the step that must come first. [Adding the high-fat part comes later, after you've conquered your sugar addiction.]

Raise Your HDL, Lower Your Triglycerides

What are HDL and triglycerides? And why should I care? Well, let's start with why you should care. It's because a low HDL number, combined with a high triglyceride number, puts you at greater risk for heart attack and stroke.

What are they? Answer: Lipoproteins (the "L" at the end of HDL and LDL), which are the body's fat transporters.

So, what's the goal here? You want to raise your good cholesterol (HDL aka high-density lipoprotein) and lower your triglycerides.

How do I fix this? Well, you've got to eat more healthy saturated fat (see my Good Fats section). But, first, you must lower your carbohydrates, which lowers your inflammation.[14]

How a Diagnosis of Metabolic Syndrome Is a Death Sentence

Whether we're aware of it or not, we're all trying to steer clear of Metabolic Syndrome, which indicates that you are at high risk for heart disease, heart attack, stroke, and other chronic diseases.

We have been misled and told that what matters most is Total Cholesterol and high LDL (aka low-density lipoprotein, aka bad cholesterol). But check out what matters most when diagnosing Metabolic Syndrome…

To be diagnosed with Metabolic Syndrome, you have to meet at least 3 of these 5 criteria:

- fat on your belly (central adiposity)

- high blood pressure

- high blood sugar

- high triglycerides

- low HDL

If high LDL matters so much, how come it didn't even make the list? So let's shine a light on what does matter most: HDL and triglycerides…

HDL - Good Cholesterol

HDL proteins transport fat out of the arteries.

Understanding what your HDL number means:

- if you're a man and your number is between 35 and 65 milligrams per deciliter (mg/dL), then you're considered "normal"; for a woman that range is 35 to 80
- less than 25, and your risk for coronary heart disease is doubled
- between 60 and 74, and your risk is "below normal"

Triglycerides

Triglycerides are, simply, fats carried in the blood.

Understanding what your triglycerides number means:

- if, after 8 hours of fasting (aka a good night's sleep), your blood test reveals your number to be less than 150 milligrams per deciliter (mg/dL), then you're considered "normal"
- 150 to 199, and you're "borderline"

- 200 to 499, and you're "high"
- 500 and higher, and you're "very high"

HDL, LDL. What's the Diff?

HDL proteins transport fat out of the arteries. LDL proteins transport fat into the arteries. It makes sense that if you've got more coming in than going out, then you're going to end up with a log jam—where your artery goes *kerplooey*! Or, as Sandy Squirrel famously says, "Did somebody say BOOM?!" just a split-second before she pushes down on the T-handle that is wired to all the dynamite on the set of the latest *Mermaid Man and Barnacle Boy* movie.

REFERENCES

1. Best anti-inflammatory – Dr. Annette Bosworth, MD. ANYWAY YOU CAN. MeTone Life, 2018, pp. 13.
2. Seizure kids – Dr. Annette Bosworth, MD. ANYWAY YOU CAN. MeTone Life, 2018, pp. 24.
3. Grocery Lists – Dr. Annette Bosworth, MD. ANYWAY YOU CAN. MeTone Life, 2018, pp. 29.
4. Grocery Lists – Dr. Ken Berry, MD. *Starting KETO: 7 Ketogenic Veggies You Can Eat as Much of as You Want!*(https://youtu.be/UsXlwieBp8I). Published by KenDBerryMD on December 28, 2017.
5. Grocery Lists – Dr. Sarah Hallberg, DO, MS, Medical Director at Virta Health (https://www.virtahealth.com/about/drsarahh allberg). *Veggies on a LCHF diet*

(https://youtu.be/YOEkQYx-ZBA). Published by FitterU on October 17, 2015.

6. No List – Dr. Annette Bosworth, MD. ANYWAY YOU CAN. MeTone Life, 2018, pp. 29.

7. No List – Dr. Sarah Hallberg, DO, MS, Medical Director at Virta Health (https://www.virtahealth.com/about/drsarahhallberg). *Veggies on a LCHF diet* (https://youtu.be/YOEkQYx-ZBA). Published by FitterU on October 17, 2015.

8. No Pills, Powders, Potions – Dr. Ken Berry, MD. *3 First Steps to Going Keto (Credit Card NOT Required)*(https://www.youtube.com/watch?v=qQQ2nwXIqzs). Published by KenDBerryMD on April 25, 2018.

9. Fructose And Fatty Liver Disease – Dr. Jason Fung, MD. THE DIABETES CODE, Chapter 7: Diabetes, a Disease of Dual Defects.

10. Walking to Lose Weight Doesn't Work – Dr. Jason Fung, MD. THE DIABETES CODE, Chapter 12: Low-Calorie Diets and Exercise: Not the Answer, The Disappointing Impact of Exercise.

11. Blood Ketones – Dr. Annette Bosworth, MD. ANYWAY YOU CAN. MeTone Life, 2018, pp. 133.

12. Diverticulitis – Dr. Ken Berry, MD. *Do Nuts and Seeds Cause Diverticulitis? Learn the Truth Behind This Common Medical Myth* (https://www.youtube.com/watch?v=8oOxNv5tLLo). Published by KenDBerryMD on October 31, 2017.
13. There Is No "Essential" Carb – Dr. Ken Berry, MD. *What is the Ketogenic Diet? (Basic Concepts Simply Discussed)* (https://youtu.be/xwKmVjSXTDk?t=74). Published by KenDBerryMD on July 17, 2018.
14. Raise Your HDL, Lower Your Triglycerides – Dr. Ken Berry, MD. *How to Raise Your HDL & Lower Your Triglycerides (NOT what you Think)* (https://www.youtube.com/watch?v=FAprJVXq1fE). Published by KenDBerryMD on August 11, 2018.

ABOUT THE AUTHOR

The last 23 years of my life have been largely defined by my looking after Mom. She was in a car accident on July 6, 1996, where she suffered a devastating brain injury. I was 24 years old at the time. She was 44. Both of our lives were, in many ways, put on hold. She and I were both released from our prisons on June 1, 2019. I hope that she is now dancing with her friends and family members who have also passed on.

During that long pause, I was mostly unemployed. I filled much of that time with computer-related projects. I repaired computers. I published a novel for a man with my late aunt. These past few years, I have published music that I myself composed, doing so under the pseudonyms of Jrex and Stu Steigmeier.

I am very proud of the albums that I have created with the help of my Korg synthesizer:

1. *Bonny & Brown (Original Soundtrack)* (https://store.cdbaby.com/cd/jrex/)

2. *Njuu Is a Great Place for Hu* (https://store.cdbaby.com/cd/jrex2/)

3. *Welcome to Weird* (https://store.cdbaby.com/cd/jrex3/)

4. *25 Hours of Hella House* (https://store.cdbaby.com/cd/jrex4/)

My favorite way to listen to my music is on Spotify. But you can find this music on every major streaming service.

That was a rather shameless plug of my other work.

I will conclude by saying that I have spent most of my life in the Piedmont region of the Deep South, about an hour south of Athens and the University of Georgia.

Made in United States
North Haven, CT
19 July 2023

39244397R00064